GW00602700

# THROUGH IT ALL

Through the Valley of Dementia
with Ron and Stella Heath
'Dad' & 'Mum' of the Torch Family

STELLA HEATH

**Distributed by**
**Shalom Christian Outreach**
**47 Stephenson Drive,**
**EAST GRINSTEAD,**
**RH19 4BG**
**Tel:01342 325105**
**Email Heathshal@aol.com**

CAMPAIGN LITERATURE
SALTCOATS

Profits from the sale of this book
will be given to regd. Christian
charities.

Published in Great Britain
by Campaign Literature

First Edition 2001


ISBN
1 872463 18 4




Printed in Great Britain
by Campaign Literature
Adelaide College
Nineyard Street
Saltcoats
Ayrshire  KA21  5HS

# THROUGH IT ALL

A Journey Through The Valley Of Dementia

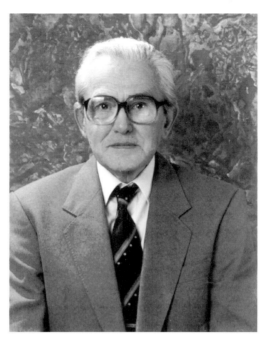

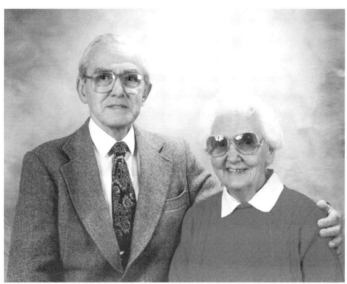

Mum and Dad — "In harness together"

# CONTENTS

# Through It All

This poem was presented to me by one of the carers.

Perhaps he's aggressive, perhaps she's rude,
Maybe they're quiet, or subdued.
You may feel nervous, or even scared,
With people whose minds are now impaired.
But before you turn to run and hide,
Look at the body with a spirit inside.

Remember the days when they could recall
Friends and family with no trouble at all.
Remember the love, the joy, the tears
Which you shared together throughout the years.
Now it's all gone, you can't have it back,
Dementia has begun its relentless attack.

Think of the families who struggle to cope
With a disease which offers so little hope.
Think of their anguish and their pain
When recognition has gone, and they try to explain,
I am your husband, I am your wife,
Together we once shared a wonderful life.

It's hard to be patient, loving and kind
To the person who has such a muddled mind.
But it's what they deserve, and what we must give
Each and every day, for as long as they live.

Anon.

# Introduction

My friend was telling me about her holiday when we were interrupted by the ringing of the telephone. When the call was over, she shook her head in frustration. "Oh dear," she sighed, "I've forgotten what I was going to say! Do you know, I'm getting worried, I keep forgetting the most simple things. You don't think my brain is going do you?"

How often we make a joke about our small lapses of memory! Usually it is the result of packing too much into our busy lives, and the simple remedy is to make a list of items to be attended to. However, sometimes we have a secret fear that the problem is more than just forgetfulness. People are becoming more aware of the value of the brain and the functions performed by it.

Brain damage is a lifelong problem to some who have suffered it at birth or because of accident or illness, and we admire those who specialise in caring for them. I have a very dear grandson who has cerebral palsy, and watching him develop has given me great admiration for those who work among folk with this handicap. But I was quite unaware of the increasing number of people (700,000 is the estimated figure currently quoted for the UK) who have developed severe brain problems, such as Alzheimer's Disease or Dementia, in some form. This usually happens later in life, though not always.

Vascular and Multi-Infarct Dementia, Alzheimer's Disease – the process of the dying of the brain – was a world far removed from my experience. I had heard the condition talked about with hushed voices and a sense of dread, and, in some cases, shame. It had never crossed my mind that I would ever be involved in this dark and little-known condition.

In this book, I feel I must open my heart to share the way the problem developed in our own family, and how by the grace of God we managed to survive the most traumatic period of my life. I do this in the hope that it will give courage to others who face similar conditions.

Although the speed of the deterioration and the character changes which come will affect sufferers differently, the stark fact of living with a precious partner and watching him "die" inside is a sorrow that is the same for us all. The way the illness affected our social life and our contact with friends and acquaintances was very difficult to live through. It was as if people were afraid to approach us, probably bewildered by the changes which the illness brought, or a feeling of inadequacy to offer the love and fellowship so sorely needed. Maybe as I share my experiences it will help to remove this barrier which prevents loving human relationships reaching those grappling with mental mysteries.

I am by nature an optimist, and in any difficulty or illness I tend to look at the light at the end of the tunnel, and endeavour to encourage the sufferers to believe things can get better. However, in common with many people, I now found myself facing an illness which is branded as "terminal". I soon became aware that Dementia of any sort is an illness for which at present there is no known solution. Terminal! What a final word! This was the first harsh fact that I had to accept when my husband's condition was diagnosed. There was no cure, just a gradual worsening of abilities and powers to think as the brain died. I found this hopeless outlook so hard to live with!

At this time I was reading the most precious Bible portion,

Psalm 23. "The Lord is my Shepherd, I shall not want". Lovely things are promised in that Psalm, with restful pastoral pictures of peace and satisfaction. But why, oh why, did David the Psalmist spoil it by putting in verse four? "Though I walk through the valley of the shadow of death". It was such a chilling contrast to the rest of the Psalm. A moment's thought made me aware that the Psalmist was being most realistic, he was writing about real life! Suddenly the words lit up. It read, "THROUGH the valley"! The Shepherd didn't leave his flock there, but led them THROUGH! There was an end in view, there was a hope after all! What is more, the verse continues, "I will fear no evil, for Thou art with me, Thy rod and Thy staff, they comfort me". There was comfort in this valley! I can't easily explain how precious these words were to me all through the traumatic period of my dear one's illness. Whatever was happening, I was not alone, the Lord WAS STILL my Shepherd!

I had several good friends who stood by me at this time. Eileen gave valuable practical help. Her mother had suffered something similar to that which Dad was going through, and she willingly helped me with the practical things which needed to be done. Sandy would phone briefly each morning to ask what sort of a night I had been having. The family were very supportive too, giving as much time as they were able from their own busy lives, and helping us with transport to hospitals and clinics. How I appreciated the way my granddaughter came to sit with her grandad for an evening early on in his illness, and played CDs to try to keep him happy. Then there was Dorothy, "The little lady at the bottom of the drive," as Dad referred to her. She was always alert to help, and many times brought Dad back from a wander in the village. There was a wealth of care in the village too, Hurstpierpoint shopkeepers, particularly, were so helpful.

## Through It All

We were often able to laugh together – not at our dear patient, we wanted above all else not to degrade him - but at the funny incidents which happened. Laughter helped us to climb over many obstacles, and soothed the soreness in our hearts which was always there. I have tried in these pages to share not only the pain, sorrow and heartache, but also the sparkles which laughter brought, and the light which illuminated a very dark pathway.

I write as it was – I can't explain everything, and I am not qualified to relate events in medical terms. I know one thing for certain – that when my faith wavered, my Shepherd was tangibly close to comfort me, even when in the darkest times I found myself unable to think, let alone to pray.

So I offer these few thoughts and experiences in the sincere hope that they may bless others who, as sufferers or carers, are going THROUGH THE VALLEY.

Stella Heath.

# CHAPTER 1
## THE COVENANT.

I have always enjoyed being busy. Sitting around doing nothing was something I found hard to do. As a child, the type of holiday spent sitting on the beach or listening silently while grown-ups talked endlessly about nothing (as I thought) was anathema to me. I usually ended up being disruptive and objectionable. I must be doing something!

When we were led by God to found and direct the work of the Torch Trust for the Blind, I became "Mum Heath" to a large family of blind and partially-sighted people all over the world. My life was crammed full of activity, and I loved it. Sometimes, it meant working through to the small hours to get things done, but I was happy and fulfilled. I loved giving all I could to the work of Torch and, more importantly, to the Lord to Whom I dedicated my life when just a girl.

For nearly forty years my husband Ron and I had worked closely together serving the Torch Family AND God had blessed us. Two houses in the UK were serving the Torch Family, fellowship groups in many towns were helping visually-impaired people at grass roots level, an orphanage and braille press was operating in Romania, and a thriving compound was functioning in Malawi. From that compound, personal and literature work was being done, coupled with practical aid to those who lacked the necessities of life, especially the visually-impaired people in Malawi and Mozambique. Also, many other countries throughout the world were being supplied with the Scriptures and Christian literature in braille. Those years had been very fruitful, and the fortieth year looked like being exciting too.

# Through It All

It was a custom of the Torch Family to hold a yearly Family Retreat – a time of re-dedication to the Lord and to the task He had given us to do. As part of our retreat, those who felt they wished to do so were invited to make a commitment using words similar to those written by John Wesley in the early days of the Methodist Church, and modified by Mr Gladstone Moore, for many years Chairman of the Torch Family.

At the Retreat, at the beginning of 1998, we were once more invited to read the words aloud together. It was always a solemn and heart-searching moment of dedication as there were some phrases which were easier to say than others.

"I am no longer my own, but Yours. Put me to what you will; rank me with whom You will; put me to doing, put me to suffering; let me be employed for You or laid aside for You; let me be full, let me be empty; let me have all things, let me have nothing; I freely and heartily yield all things to Your pleasure and disposal. And now, O glorious and blessed God, Father, Son and Holy Spirit, You are mine, and I am yours. So be it. And the covenant which I have made on earth, let it be ratified in Heaven. Amen."

My personal reactions to the Covenant were mixed. "Put me to doing" – that suited me fine. I was all set, looking forward to more years of active service.
"Put me to suffering" – not so good! Suffering had come our way in many forms in the past, but we always hoped we would have no more!
"Let me be employed" – oh yes, indeed!

"OR LAID ASIDE FOR YOU" – oh, that was something I hoped would never happen!

But it did!

As a couple, we were all set for a great leap forward, serving at the special exhibitions, speaking at the rallies, and letting the needs of visually-impaired people be known. I enjoyed the planning stage, and was looking forward happily to the part Ron and I would be able to play. Forty great years indeed! The year 1999 was going to be the best yet – or so we thought!

I had just completed writing a short history, describing events during those 40 years, when I began to realise that all was not well.

Even as I was working on the proofs of the book, and helping to plan the displays, I noticed a slight change in Ron, the dear Dad Heath of the Torch Family. It was as if we could both sense the shadows of a dark valley lying in the path before us, and little chilly winds would blow from it, making us wonder if we would be able to fulfil our role in the celebrations after all.

# Through It All

# Chapter 2
# Father Of Four, Dad To Many.

The noise level in the dining-room at Torch House had reached a crescendo. As staff and helpers came in to dinner, they were laughing and sharing their experiences of the morning's work. The noise was deafening! Suddenly Dad Heath's voice rose above the din.

"Can I have a bit of quiet, please!"

Immediately there was silence. Then Dad Heath reverently led the family in grateful thanks to God for the food that was about to be served.

But Dad Heath rarely raised his voice. He was the meekest of men, never pushing himself forward, or forcing others to accept his opinions. He was respected by all who worked with him. His honesty and sincerity, combined with fairness and a willingness to listen, had earned him that respect through the years during which he had served the Torch Family as Dad. He occasionally made mistakes, of course, but was not too proud to say "sorry", and his wise counsel, when problems arose, was a valued contribution to the well-being and growth of the Torch Family world-wide.

For 39 years he had given his time and energy to the welfare of visually-impaired people. Through many hard times, many late nights, many perplexing problems, he had kept a steadying hand on the tiller as he piloted the boat through the storms that inevitably arose.

Faith in God was something that had grown in him since babyhood. As a little boy he was afraid of dogs, and the

11

family love to tell the story of how one morning he sat at the top of the stairs afraid to come down. As he waited, he sang, "I will trust, I will trust, and not be afraid," then he stopped and shouted, "Daddy, is the dog tied up?" Even young as he was, faith and action went together!

This element of believing faith was just what was needed in the early days when the Torch Family was developing. As husband and wife we were led to initiate a number of far-reaching projects. I might have had the inspiration, but Dad Heath had the commonsense to test them and then help them forward. His motto was, "Prayer first, action later. If a project is of God, then He will meet every need. If not, we don't want it!"

One of Dad's frequently used phrases was, "It all needs to start with prayer." When he was showing people round the house and works, he would always say, "Everything you see here in Torch is a miracle, because it is an answer to prayer." Prayer certainly played a very important part in his life, a legacy which has been handed down to others.

"Prayer first, words and actions afterwards" was his way of conducting business, making decisions and coping with problems.

Sometimes we failed to take enough heed of his warnings, they were so gently given. I remember his plea for the family to avoid destructive criticism, and instead to encourage even those who were struggling. Many pitfalls could have been avoided if we had all taken that warning to heart.

However, his role as Dad of the Torch Family was not his only one. He was also father to four of his own natural children. He was strict but loving, and tender and sympathetic to all who were in pain. He was always the gentleman and taught his children to be courteous as well. In those days we had no car, so we would walk miles when on holiday, a pastime not completely to the liking of his children! We used to have railway camping coach holidays, when he would cheerfully fetch water, fill the stove with oil, and even cook some of the meals. We sometimes went boating, though "ON the water, but not IN it" was father's motto. Only once did he voluntarily go into the water when the children were young and that was when we were walking on the beach in Brighton, and Philip, usually the one who dared to take risks, ran into the sea, and was caught by a large wave. Without a moment's hesitation, distaste for water forgotten, father ran through the waves, grabbed Philip's jacket, and rescued him. Soaked to the skin on a raw February day, we went into a café and dried them both there.

The only other times when he had to overcome his dislike for water and getting wet was when over the years a considerable number of visitors to Torch House asked him to baptise them in the swimming pool at Hallaton. His face showed how much he disliked the water, but he fulfilled his role with dignity and indeed with great joy. It was a real sorrow when the three young men of the Ferraby family asked him to baptise them, and he was far too ill to do it. He had watched the family growing up from birth, and would have loved to have officiated on that occasion.

He is remembered too for the sense of quiet devotion he brought to the communion services that were regularly held at Torch House. Many people were blessed by those times when we felt very near to the Lord.

And then, after almost forty years of service, we were all set to celebrate the amazing way in which the Torch Family

D

had grown. Dad and I were due to be part of that celebration.

Would it have been all to the glory of God? Or would a little of the glory have gone astray and been directed at us? We don't know, but God in His wisdom closed the door on us being part of the programme, and as Dad Heath said repeatedly, "God's will must be put first always!"

Sometimes, the will of God seems to be enshrouded in mystery, and so hard to understand. That is when we are tempted to ask, "Why?" One day there will be no "why?" but, instead, the exclamation, "My! I didn't know God had THIS in store for me!"

"No discipline seems pleasant at the time, but painful. Later on, however, it produces a harvest of righteousness and peace for those who have been trained by it." Hebrews 12:11.

# Chapter 3
## Bruges.

As I look back and view the chequered pathway of 1998-1999 there are some things which amaze me. Before we had any real idea of the immensity of the problems ahead of us, God had prepared a little surprise for Ron.

We decided to use an accumulation of air miles to go on a trip by Eurostar through the Channel tunnel for four nights in Belgium. Ron was unusually enthusiastic about this holiday. Normally he went on holiday not because he wanted to, but because he wanted to give me a break from routine.

I had realised by this time that I would have to take charge of the tickets, and arrange our trip throughout. It gave me a pang of regret to see the frustration evident in Ron as he saw me doing what he had always done so well. But it was obvious that I could no longer rely on him to be the tower of strength he had always been on holiday.

All went smoothly, and we enjoyed the effortless journey across the Channel. I managed to hire a taxi, and we were soon settled in our hotel room. The strange environment proved a problem from the first to Ron, and I had to lead him to the dining-room and show him the way to the toilet several times before he was settled enough to begin to enjoy the holiday.

We explored Brussels, which was beautiful and interesting. Then we decided to spend a day in Bruges. What a lovely place it was! Even though the weather was unsettled we were able to have a peaceful trip up the canal system to see Bruges from the water. We visited the lace-makers, and marvelled at their dexterity. We visited some of the little shops around the tourist area. Then we walked into the main part of the town to see some of the famous churches.

I confess this was not something that brought me a great deal of delight, and after we had looked round three or four of them I was wanting to get back to the lace-makers. However, Ron decided to go to another – I can't remember its name – where he became very interested in the murals which were painted all round the church. It was rather gloomy inside, and I looked longingly through the door to the sunshine outside. Ron stood for a long time staring at a mural depicting Christ stumbling beneath the weight of the Cross. Eventually, he moved through the doorway into the street.

"I've met with God in there!" he said, his voice full of wonder. "In that church, I heard Him speak to me. He said, 'I did this for you!' He spoke to me!" Ron's face was alight as I had seldom seen it. Something very real had happened. He had met with the Lord!

Over the next few weeks, wherever he could, he told the story of his encounter with God in that church. The experience had brought a lot of joy and peace to his heart.

Over the years of our life together, people of all ages would share with us their own personal walk with the Lord. Some had known a blinding sense of the majesty of God with experiences of overwhelming joy. I could readily relate to such touches from God, for they were like those I had realised myself when I gave my life to the Lord as an eight-year old. The memory of that moment is still as vivid now as it was then. There were other people who came to chat with us who were not able to recount such an experience, although they knew they were truly born into the family of God. We used to comment on the fact that Ron could identify with the latter group, whereas I could identify with the former, so between us we could be of some help to both.

But now, as we began to enter the dark valley, though we had no idea how dark it would be, the Lord had reached down and whispered a personal assurance to His child, one which would be so sorely needed in future days.

I would have said that Ron would never be moved by art in that particular form, in fact neither of us would have thought a picture on a wall could so profoundly move us. It has shown me how very big is the God we serve, big enough to use anything, anywhere, at any time, when He wants to comfort and fortify His children.

"I did it for you!" Even now the words bring a sense of awe to my own heart as they did to Ron in that church in Bruges.

# Through It All

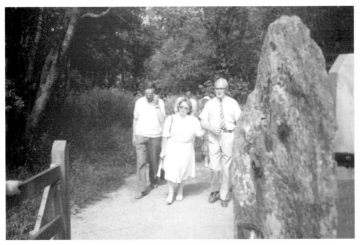

Dad Heath in the Lake District
Always willing to lend his arm to any visually-impaired people
and take them for a walk

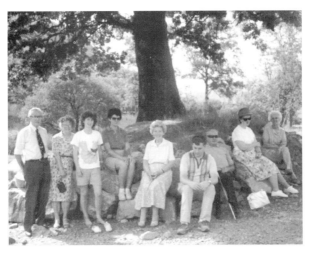

Time for a short rest — Taking a group for a walk was
something Dad loved to do

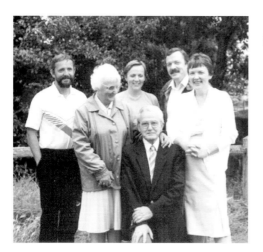

The family —
Sapphire wedding
1988

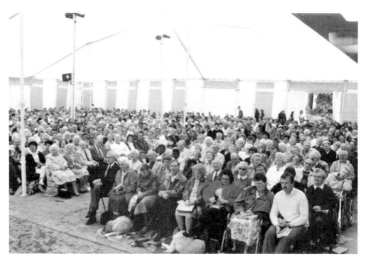

At Keswick 1991
On the front row with guide dogs and members of the
houseparty

# Chapter 4
# Chill Winds.

It was part-way through the summer of 1998 that I began to notice that Ron was finding simple jobs like carpentry almost too difficult to cope with. He had always been a great do-it-yourself man, and had tackled some very ambitious projects successfully. But now he found it so hard to fix a shelf safely, and had great difficulty in getting it straight. He easily lost his way too, especially when driving. Other signs began to show that something was wrong. He complained occasionally of headaches, "it's as if I've got a skull cap on that is too tight," he would say. "But it's nothing! Don't worry, it will pass!" We visited the doctor, but apart from a small blood pressure problem, there seemed no cause for alarm.

After 55 years of marriage we were well used to each other's methods and moods, idiosyncrasies and quirks – not that there were many – our married life was a good one, in which we were one in purpose. In fact, decision making was so mutual that we didn't need to devote time to great discussions before making up our minds, we would know the way we were both thinking. So, when the first signs of something wrong began to show in his behaviour, it was hard to understand.

A few of our friends began to notice his failing mental capacity, though most people didn't know that anything was wrong until some months later.

The realisation hit me when we were out shopping. I had noticed that Ron was having difficulty with figures, frequently forgetting his pin number and having other small lapses of memory. That day we were shopping for small odds and ends, and I think we had gone into a shop to buy some batteries. The purchase cost about £1.50. Ron smiled sweetly at the assistant as he paid her, and then pressed a ten pound note into her hand.

She was astounded. "Oh, no!" she said, embarrassed. "I can't..."

"Of course you can," Ron replied, with such a firm voice that the girl stammered her thanks and disappeared behind the counter.

Outside the shop I remonstrated with him. "Ron, you shouldn't have given so much to the assistant!" I said, "We can't afford to tip like that with every purchase!"

Ron shrugged his shoulders. "It's all right. She had a nice smile!"

This was so completely out of character; I could hardly believe that my dear cautious banker was throwing money away like that!

I became even more concerned when I noticed other evidences of mistakes with finances. I found outstanding bills which had been covered over by a pile of other correspondence and left unpaid until red reminders came. Ron spent hours trying to work out simple calculations when his bank statement came. It was obvious he was finding figure-work too difficult.

Another difficulty which arose at this time was when Ron was leading meetings. He would choose the same hymn twice, and be oblivious to the remarks of the congregation. When recounting the history of the growth of the Torch Family, he would say something quite inaccurate, even ludicrous, like, "It all began seven months ago when we had a blind girl to tea." I began to feel tense and anxious every time he spoke. He was, however, thoroughly at home when taking the Communion worship at Torch House. Few things went wrong there, as we concentrated on the remembrance of the Lord's suffering and death.

What could I do in this situation? I must do something about the finances or we would get into debt, and, for everyone's sake, something needed to be done about this inability to take meetings. I felt I was walking a tightrope. Ron had always dealt with financial matters, and would not let me handle any of them. "You have other things to do," he always said. How was I going to take over now, and play my part in steering us through this time? It was so hard to get the balance. I wanted to let Ron still feel he was the man in charge, and to preserve his sense of dignity, yet at the same time we had to find the right solution to these problems. The trouble was that Ron didn't seem to recognise that anything was wrong.

Something would have to be done, and soon!

As the clouds began to gather, my precious Psalm meant more and more to me. My Shepherd would show me the way.

# Through It All

# CHAPTER 5
## DIAGNOSIS.

We had adjusted our routine to cope with the changes that were necessary. I had managed to come to terms with the finances; Dad was finding life difficult as he had to admit there were things he could no longer do; but we were able to share these problems, and talking together helped us to understand each other. He kept asking if we could go back to Bruges, but I felt unable to take the risk, as he tended to wander off and get lost more frequently now. I think if we had revisited the city it would probably have been an anticlimax, so I tried to use tapes to satisfy his spiritual needs with varying success. However, he always responded when the Scriptures were read to him.

Understanding some of Dad's reactions was not easy at first; we had to learn to take each turn of events as it came along. We were entering another phase of our journey through the valley, as the disease developed. Now, other things were starting to go wrong with Dad's body. The first intimation of this new phase came when we were having a pleasant meal with Florence and Michael Jay. Suddenly Dad put his knife and fork down and said, "This is it!" We all looked at him, wondering what he meant. "I've just lost the sight in my right eye!" he said.

We went to the doctor who referred us to an eye clinic in Brighton. Ron was tested thoroughly but there was nothing much to account for the loss of sight, except that he had an unusual blood count that he had lived with for a long time. Then, just as suddenly, the sight came back in his right eye. We breathed a sigh of relief. "Just a passing problem," we thought.

But things were by no means right. At a restaurant soon afterwards, Dad suddenly stopped as he was eating his dessert, with spoon poised in mid-air. He sat motionless for several minutes, then blinked, and continued eating. What had gone wrong now? I concluded it must have been some sort of mini-stroke. Another visit to the doctor resulted in arrangements being made for a series of tests in the local hospital.

Then alarm bells rang loudly in my head when the next physical symptom occurred. We were on an Outreach in Cheam, accompanying the Team as they ministered at an Old People's Club. Sandy was singing and David and Trevor were playing their instruments. We had, in fact, just finished and were preparing to leave, when suddenly Dad collapsed in a heap on the floor. For a few moments he made no movement, and I thought he had passed away, but then he opened his eyes and tried to sit up. Ambulance men were called, and they lifted him into a chair. As we were due to have tests at the local hospital the next day, he was allowed to go home. Was this another mini-stroke?

We tried to live as normally as was possible. In his usual helpful way, Dad tried to continue those little chores which he had done for many years, like bringing a cup of tea to me before I dressed in the morning.

Oh dear! The problems we had with that simple task! Dad's body clock went wrong, and he would wake me up at 2.30 am, or some other unmentionable hour, with a cup of tea. He would get up himself at 4 or 5 am, and want to go to bed at 7pm. Then, very early one morning, he came in to me and said, "I can't get the kettle to boil, I know I've switched it on!" I staggered out of bed and went to the kitchen. He had switched on the electric mixer instead of the kettle! So I bought a bright green kettle, the colour really hit you in the eye! However, he still couldn't get the right appliance switched on, so I suggested I didn't really need a cup of tea in bed! Nothing daunted, still trying to be helpful, he brought me a bowl of prunes and sweetcorn for my breakfast. I could have wept! He was determined to do the little things he had always done to show he cared, but now, whatever he tried to do went wrong.

He took to spending an hour at a time wrapped in thought. I well remember one occasion when he came to me and said, "I've been thinking."

"What about, dear?" I asked.

"Well," he said, very solemnly, "I do hope you will agree with my decision, but I have decided we ought not to have any more children." As he was 84, and I was nearly 80, I agreed without question. Visions of Sarah and Abram flitted into my mind. I had to go away and indulge in a hearty laugh! Dear Dad's mind was obviously going back to earlier years when such a decision might well have been necessary.

Meanwhile, the hospital tests had to be worked through. He was interested in them all. The only one he had problems with was the one that recorded his heartbeat for twenty-four hours. For this he had to have a tape recorder strapped to him for a whole day and night, with terminals fastened to his chest. My! How we managed to get a reading of his heartbeat from that I don't know, as I was constantly having to reconnect some of the terminals which had worked loose. Night time was not too difficult, as fortunately he didn't fidget in bed, but at one point during the day the whole rather bulky tape recorder slipped and fell to the ground. He looked so crestfallen, as if it was his fault that it had happened. I laughed; "Oh dear," I said, "now ALL the terminals have come loose. How shall I know which goes where? Suppose I fix it so that you have a recording that is back to front!" We both had to smile. I fastened the clumsy contraption to his waist, so that he looked as if he had suddenly put on weight. At least I made sure it was secure this time! Fortunately, I must have put the plugs into the right sockets, for he didn't have to go through that process again.

We went to the doctor to find out the results of the tests. He chatted a little to Dad, then he handed me a piece of paper with one word written on it. "DEMENTIA". I winced. It seemed such a cruel word, and I was so glad the doctor had not said it aloud. All the way through this experience he was so very understanding and helpful. He put us in touch with the welfare department that dealt specially with this particular problem. But that word haunted me in the days to come! The chill winds from the valley were beginning to be felt! We were finding out practically what might be in store.

There were times when laughter came to the rescue. Dad began to hide things in unlikely places. I would find articles like cloth serviettes, even cutlery, protruding from his pockets, or hidden under the cushion of his chair, even thrown in the bin! A plate of cakes prepared for a visitor had disappeared. Eileen was with me by this time, and together we searched and searched to try to find it.

"Strange," said Eileen, "I can't think of another place to look. I've checked the dishwasher, where I found a pint of milk the other day. I've looked in the refrigerator, and even the washing machine, but there is no sign anywhere of that plate of cakes!" Weeks later we found it, when all the cakes had grown furry coats, in the airing cupboard! We just had to laugh!

A new suite of furniture arrived when I was out shopping. Dad insisted that it was not complete, though the three pieces were there as large as life. He became quite unreasonable about this and we had to pacify the men who brought it. I must say they were very helpful when they realised the problem. This was the first time that people outside the immediate circle of home had been aware that something was wrong with Dad. I had an urge to shield him from the world outside our home, for so many people have strange ideas about any affliction involving the brain and mind. I wanted friends to visualise him as the dear, gentle man he had always been, so I worked hard to keep him looking smart and normal.

But the relentless progress of the dementia went on, and I had to adapt to the changes it brought. I had to make sure that I repeated any instruction I gave at least twice; it was as if it would not register in Dad's mind unless I repeated it. Though I knew little about the illness, I could see that the disease was progressing, as the medical people warned me it would.

Eventually, welfare visitors spent time explaining more about the progress of the illness, and it did help; though the first time I was put in the picture I felt weak at the knees! I was always glad that it was John Baigent, a dear Christian doctor, who was the first one to take me aside and explain in greater detail what lay before us. He said, "Stella, your dear husband will die. There is no cure for dementia of this sort. He will eventually become helpless as a baby. Don't make the mistake of trying to look after him when he becomes worse. It will be more than is possible in a home situation." His concern and his prayers were a great strength to me, and they continued through all the stages of Dad's illness. Such friendship was so valuable at this stage. I had been troubled by advice from some of my friends who told me I must never let him go into a nursing home, that I was to remember how good he had been to me, and I should keep him with me all the time, come what may, as they had done when their own husbands were dying. I had been very willing to keep Ron, whatever, but later, when the strain became intolerable, I was comforted to think back to Dr John's words. My friends' husbands did not have dementia.

On our last visit to the doctor, he had told Dad firmly that he was not under any circumstance to drive!

"The doctor has said that I mustn't drive long distances any more," he told the family.

"He said you were not under ANY circumstances to drive at all!" I retorted. "And I've got the car keys!"

"But I enjoy driving!" he said sadly, like a child who was being denied a favourite toy. I was more than glad to hide the keys as I had suffered many nightmarish occasions as a passenger in recent trips, when only the good hand of the Lord spared us from being involved in dreadful accidents.

I had a wonderful answer to prayer at this time, as I was not able to drive the large Astra, the car which we had used for years. Some friends asked me if I was interested in a smaller car. I said that I was. They told me of a neat little Rover Metro with only 7,000 miles on the clock, going for a very reasonable sum. I felt at once that this was God's provision to help us to keep mobile. This was important when we were still having to visit hospitals, respite homes and day centres.

Gradually, we were managing to adjust to the changes that became necessary, as the disease relentlessly continued to alter dear Dad's personality.

# Chapter 6
# Dad? Talkative?

The progress of Ron's illness was now reaching the stage where we were seeing frequent character changes. I hesitated about writing an account of these, and the rest of our journey through the valley of death, because of the pain experienced by us all. But it would not be a true picture of the whole of the Good Shepherd's care and leading if we failed to show the rough places as they were.

Those carers who are treading a similar pathway will be able to relate to the dragging weariness, the feeling of having lost one's identity in a sea of pressure and pain, and becoming a rather inefficient robot instead of a human being. The inability to pray for any length of time, through sheer exhaustion, was at first a shock. Praying at times seemed to be impossible. But, above the feeling of numbness, of wondering if I'd ever cope, came sweet little touches from God Himself. A card with a loving message on it; a phone call, brief and to the point, assuring of prayer, meant so much to me. It seemed that other Christians were being commissioned by God to pray when I couldn't. The wonder of the Family of God was precious at this time. I am sure that similar experiences to these are shared by many carers throughout our world.

Inexorably, the deterioration in Ron seemed to escalate, and the once quiet, gentle, self-effacing man we all knew and loved became gregarious, assertive, and talking at most inappropriate times about nothing which made sense. I noticed other distinct changes in Ron's behaviour as well at this time.

We had some embarrassing moments when Ron would

blurt out something which could be taken the wrong way. What he said at these times in no way reflected his true thinking. I had met enough friends suffering from forms of brain damage to be able to see straightaway that Ron's remarks had bypassed his normal brain control system. This was evident when Ron's sister Doris came to take him for a walk. I was always glad to see her, as she brought a sense of normality to our day. Her visits gave a measure of relief to Ron. She even had some success in engaging in a few quite rational scraps of conversation with him. Doris lives with her sister Elma, who is unable to go out at all, but whose prayer ministry is valued greatly by all who know her.

Doris passed on a cheery message from Elma to Ron, but to our surprise he retorted, "Tell her to mind her own business!" At first I felt embarrassed, I was anxious that no-one would be hurt, as that was a way of talking which Ron would never indulge in. I was gratified to see that everyone treated it as a joke. To Ron it was a cliché that he must have heard many times, but was certainly not in the habit of using. We began to experience other occasions when Ron spoke in a way that he would never have spoken when rational. This phase of Ron's illness brought a complete reversal to our pattern for living. In the past, I had usually been the one who had to try to keep conversation going, and I used to have difficulty in drawing Ron into making his contribution. Now, I found myself having to try to curb his flow of words.

I first encountered this embarrassing urge which Ron had when some visitors came to lunch. The meal was all ready, the guests were seated, and I asked Ron to give thanks for the food. He did, in a very muddled sort of way which was impossible to follow. But I realised with horror that he didn't seem to know when to stop. After fifteen minutes, by which time the vegetables were getting cold, I got up from the table and whispered, "Thanks dear, but that's enough!" Even then he was not keen to stop. How I hated having to say this to him! But his prayers were so jumbled up that it was impossible for us to follow them.

I will never forget a visit we made to a Garden Centre. We were sitting waiting for a cream tea which we had ordered. Ron usually liked going to such places, and it seemed to relax him. But this time he was fidgeting about as if searching for something.

"What do you want dear?" I said. "Be patient, they will be coming to serve us quite soon!" I thought he was getting tired of waiting for his cream tea.

"I haven't got my Bible!" he said, patting his pocket where he sometimes kept a small Testament.

"But you don't need a Bible to eat a cream tea," I said, rather puzzled.

He cleared his throat and started to get to his feet. Immediately I realised that he was intending to deliver a sermon to the other people enjoying their cream tea. The trouble was that I knew he would not be able to say even one sentence which would make sense. I quickly grabbed the nearest part of him, which happened to be his braces, and pulled him back into his chair.

"Sit down," I ordered. "This is no place for a sermon!"

I'm afraid he was very angry with me because I had hindered him from speaking. I had noticed that he was becoming more and more intolerant of any interruption when he had made up his mind to talk. What a change this was! Having spent many years trying to encourage Ron to speak I now had to be the one to prevent him from speaking. He used to like to go to the little church at the end of the drive in Hurstpierpoint some evenings, and he received a very warm welcome there. However, the dear people did have moments when his yen for speaking disrupted their worship. They were so very Christlike, gentle and patient with him. I did appreciate their attitude.

A dear friend, known to us for many years, had passed away, and I longed to go to the funeral. I thought perhaps it would be an occasion when Ron would not be so disruptive. I knew that if he had been well he would have made every effort to go to this particular funeral. So, I decided to risk it and go.

"I want my Bible!" Ron demanded just before we started.

"Ron, you won't need your Bible this time, just listen like the rest of us!" I didn't want to take too many pieces of baggage which could "stray", as Ron did put things in strange places at times.

All went well, although conversation with old friends was painful at times, but altogether we met with understanding and love. Two days later, I was checking Ron's jacket ready to take it to the cleaners, when I discovered, in his pocket, three pages torn from his Bible. They had come from John chapters 2 and 3. He was determined to be ready to preach on that occasion. As I had said no to him taking a Bible, he tore out the pages instead. He would make sure he was ready.

Many times in the past we had visited fellowship groups and churches where Ron had been asked to speak, sometimes without warning. Some part of his memory had made him want to be prepared in case he should be asked to give a talk at the funeral.

Visitors were few by this time, which was understandable, as his talkative behaviour puzzled them. The changes in his nature were so much more evident now, and some of our friends could not take it. Sandy came to see him one day. He seemed to know her, probably because she was blind. But he had made up his mind that the young man who had kindly brought her down from Crawley was the doctor.

"I'm not the doctor," the young man stammered, looking most embarrassed. Dad took no notice, and began to talk about his medical problems in detail, which totally confused our visitor. Following his reasoning as he rambled on was increasingly difficult, and in the end impossible.

By now Eileen had come to join me, and as there were times when Little Torch was full up for houseparties, Eileen made up a bed-settee each night in the lounge. This proved to be a life-saver on several occasions. The help Eileen gave was so quietly unobtrusive, but so practical. As the trek through the valley of dementia grew harder I do not know how I could have managed without her help. Her self-appointed task was to cope with the laundry, which was an increasing chore. It seemed that the washing machine was working all day.

One night I went to bed at around 11pm after making sure Ron had all he needed. He seemed extra alert, and sat up in bed talking away about nothing, hardly waiting to take a breath. I tried to settle down for the night, hoping for a little sleep. Still he talked.

"Ron dear, it's late, and I'm tired, please settle down and

go to sleep!" I said.

There was no response at all to this, just a torrent of unrelated words, going on endlessly in spite of my plea for quiet. Suddenly the bedroom door opened, and Eileen walked in.

"Dad, will you please be quiet, I can't get to sleep because you are making so much noise!"

Instantly he lay down, and blissful silence reigned. I had been warned by my medical friends that there would be times when he would "play up" with me, but behave well, even charmingly, with other people. I was thankful that Eileen was within earshot.

I looked at Ron as he slept and wondered what had happened, and what was still happening inside that dear head. What were his feelings? His frustrations were evident, and his bewilderment was painful to watch. What imbalance was it that had changed him so drastically?

Around this time, Ron took to getting out of bed in the middle of the night. His one aim seemed to be to go out of the bedroom and to wander into the main house at Little Torch. The only thing to stop him was a fire door, which must not be locked. If he had roamed round at night in the house it could have frightened the guests badly. This meant that he had to be watched all the time. I learned to sleep with one ear cocked to try to restrain him the moment he stirred. He rebelled quite vehemently when he was prevented from leaving the bedroom, and as it took as long as thirty minutes to get him to go back to bed, I would rouse up at the slightest movement and do my best to prevent him from getting up. Sometimes I was successful, sometimes not.

These night-time battles were the occasions when Ron was most aggressive. Dear darling man, he would never ever hurt anyone, yet at these times he would grab me in real anger, and I had difficulty sometimes to get free from his grasp. When he gripped my arms or hands I could manage, but I dreaded him clutching at my neck. I was so glad to be able to call for assistance if things became too bad.

My brother and sister-in-law came to be with me when Eileen went on holiday. One night, I didn't hear the first stirrings as Ron swung out of bed, and he was soon in full spate, demanding to go out. Try as I would, I couldn't make him get back into bed, and after struggling for about forty five minutes, I called for help. The moment he heard Bernard's voice he responded, and meekly got into bed. I was so grateful for the help I received from friends and family at this time. I thanked the Lord every day for them all.

There was one small glimpse into the real, loving husband who was fast disappearing from my life. It happened one night when I had a touch of pleurisy, and wanted to curl up with a hot bottle to get some comfort. Ron had other ideas, he started to get out of bed and was very angry when I begged him to settle down.

"Oh dear," I sighed in desperation. "I wish you'd settle dear, I don't feel at all well, and I'm longing to get back into bed. Please swing your legs up on the bed and I'll tuck you in."

"No!" he cried emphatically.

I cried to God to make a miracle happen as that night I had no human handy to call upon. Suddenly, he climbed back into bed, and was asleep in a few minutes. Next morning, as I was preparing the routine of medicines, clothing and protective pads ready for when he woke up, he stirred in the bed and said, "Well, how is your pain today?" I can't tell you how overjoyed I was to know that the dear caring man I thought I had lost altogether was still there, and somewhere, under all the confusion, he had remembered that I wasn't well.

# Chapter 7
## Medication

There are many issues which are the subject of debate concerning the ethics of medical treatment to sustain life. Normally, they are on the fringe of our experience and rarely occupy any great place in our thinking. But those very issues can become all-important when illness strikes a loved one. Problems such as when to use life-support machines, or to administer costly drugs, or take other steps, often painful, in an effort to prolong life, seem to be remote from our experience. Then, suddenly, they take on a much greater urgency when we are faced with those very situations ourselves. The issue of euthanasia, active or passive, has a new poignancy when watching a member of one's own family suffering. The use of drugs to maintain existence, alleviate suffering, comfort the dying, prolong life, now become matters requiring personal consideration and decision.

I looked across at Ron's sleeping form; he seemed so peaceful that night. I knew that the reason was because the sleeping tablets were doing their work and I was relieved. Maybe I'd be able to get a few hours sleep as a result.

But was it right that he should be so doped just to give me some sleep? And what about all the other pills, which at one point amounted to 18 a day? What were the reasons for giving them to him? What about the tremendous expense this must be to the NHS and to what purpose?

The whole question of Ron's medication troubled me. At what point do we have to choose between artificially prolonging a life that holds nothing but anguish, and allowing nature to take its own course?

We had occasionally discussed this very matter together in better times. Ron had always felt that as a Christian he would rather not be hindered in his journey to be with Christ. He had said that he didn't want to be kept alive by mechanical means or medication beyond what was needed to give comfort during the natural process of dying.

But what were we doing now? A pill to help his blood to circulate, a pill to alleviate the brain anguish he was suffering, a pill to help with the restlessness that at one stage characterised every waking moment, a pill for...what WERE all the pills for?

I asked a few questions, and was assured that none of them were given to prolong his life unnaturally, but rather to make it more bearable. That last aim was not being reached, as his waking moments were devoid of all natural enjoyment. I did assure myself, however, that none of his medication was unduly prolonging his life.

I sat on the bed and watched him as he lay asleep, and I felt a wave of guilt to think that I had been so cold and calculating about his pills. "Oh Ron, I want you back so badly. I don't want you to die, but I can't bear this living death that you are enduring!" Choosing the right medication must present a constant problem to the medical profession. Some of the drugs used now are very expensive. Was there anything Ron was taking which was not needed? Periodically, I talked with the doctor or nurse, and some of his many pills were discontinued without any noticeable effect. The fact remained that all they could do was to make Ron as comfortable as possible while the brain-death took its relentless course. The word "incurable" is a very hard one to face.

We had shared 55 years of happy marriage, when Ron had been the gentle guide and protector which I so needed. Together we had seen God do wonderful, miraculous things, and my postbag was full of letters from lovely, grateful people who felt that we had brought life to them in establishing the Torch Family, and bringing them to Christ. But now, there he lay, my other half; closer even than mother or father, son or daughter, going through the agony of a changed personality, easily provoked, angry at times, even telling me to go away. Part of me was dying with him.

In the end the medication problem was resolved. As a Christian I believed in the sanctity of life. We would only use drugs to ease the pain and anguish as Ron's illness progressed. Life and death are in the hands of the Lord. He Who knew the path before us had promised he would never leave us in the lurch. He would carry us through; yes, THROUGH this valley, to something so much richer and more glorious than anything we had experienced before. For Ron, the gates of the City were within sight. He loved the Lord and he wanted to be with Him. For me, I would have more opportunities to prove Him as my Shepherd as I continued to serve Him.

I was at this time facing other anxieties of a different nature, when it became necessary for us to move from the annex at Little Torch. The old house had to be emptied for essential improvements, so our accommodation was needed to house the dear little family who were living there. At no time did they put any pressure on us, in fact they were so gentle and prayerful as they discussed the necessary plans and alterations for the future of the work.

We had always understood that, should the time come when we had to move from the annex, the Torch Family would be able to give us help to find another home. We had originally given the proceeds from the sale of our home to provide the Torch Family with the first Torch House. We had also spent a considerable sum helping to build and equip a bungalow in the grounds of the house in Hallaton, thus using up all our assets. We, and the Torch Council, were shocked to discover that as we had been trustees we were not able to benefit by one penny from the Trust. There were many suggestions offered by well-meaning people to try to overcome this problem. However, the Torch Council could not see their way clear to take any of them up, as there was a welter of red tape and many legal snags in the way. We were cast on the One Who had our lives in His hand. His promises in that wonderful Psalm 23 were still there.

Ron was aware of the housing problem, and at first it disturbed him. But as the disease progressed, it faded from his mind, though he pleaded with me repeatedly to buy the tickets to take him on the train to "home". I never did discover where "home" was. Increasingly, Ron was taking refuge in sleep. "It's nice to sleep," he said, "the confusion stops when I'm asleep!"

We were entering a very painful phase for sufferer and carer alike, for Ron was spending much of his time head in hands, sobbing out prayers to the Lord to help him. He was suffering increasing pain and anguish, and none of the pills seemed to help, except those which sent him to sleep. It was so distressing to witness this agony. In more lucid moments he tried to describe it as like being drawn into a terrible black pit that was all confusion, despair and doubt. Nothing seemed to relieve it, except about five minutes of reading from the Scriptures, after which it all flooded back again.

He couldn't tolerate music at all, even the type he used to enjoy. One day I was busy in the kitchen, having settled Ron with a very restful gardening programme on the TV. Without my realising it, the adverts had come on, and were particularly strident. When I went into the room the TV was dead.

"It was nasty!" Ron exclaimed, "So I stopped it!" He couldn't find out how to work either the remote control or the switch on the TV, so he had torn the connection to the aerial from the wall.

Perhaps there was something to be said for sleeping pills!

# Through It All

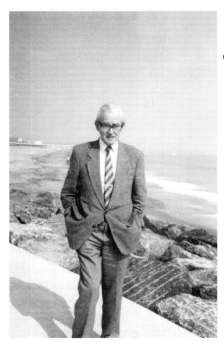

Oh, I do like to be
beside the
seaside!

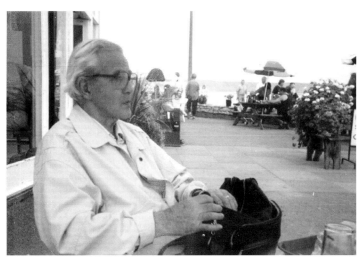

Dad Heath at the seaside — Taking care of the baggage while
the rest of the party went for a swim

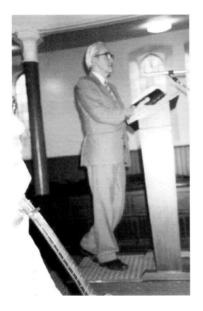

This is rather a hazy
picture but *so* typical of
Dad Heath sharing the
Scriptures in church

Malawi 1993
Dad Heath has a friendly
chat with Jonah, a blind
member of the Malawi
Council, and with one of
the workers at the Sazdla
Torch Fellowship

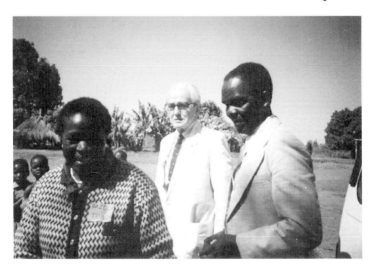

# Chapter 8
# Wanderlust

One of the early symptoms which showed in Ron's life-style was an urge to go out. He used to make trips to the village of Hurstpierpoint at every opportunity. I encouraged these little walks as it seemed a harmless way to get exercise. One day he said that he wanted to go to the Mint House, a very nice stationer's shop in the High Street which was about five minutes walk away. After he had been away nearly an hour I began to get worried, especially as a neighbour had remarked that he was not always too careful when crossing the road. I rang up a friend who lives on the High Street, but she had not seen or heard anything which might give us a clue. I began to get really worried, as it was beginning to get dark. Two of our dear friends, Gail and Lilian, who were both at Little Torch at the time, took their car and scoured the village. There was no sign of Ron. They turned towards Hassocks. Soon they spotted him striding out along the mile and a half of road without a care in the world!

"Where HAVE you been?" I asked, anxiety making me sound rather sharp.

"I've had a nice walk," he smiled. "I looked for the shop but couldn't find it, so I had a little wander round instead." He had evidently become disorientated at the end of the drive and turned right instead of left. We all sighed with relief, but I began to wonder how much longer I could let him wander freely.

The disorientation became worse, and his little excursions to the village had to be taken with an escort. Some days he would become so restless that he would demand walks every half-hour or so. This taxed me considerably, and were it not for the help of Eileen who came alongside to help me I would not have managed to keep up with the daily chores like washing and cleaning, chores which were getting heavier as we tried to cope with the illness.

The welfare and social services were helpful. They arranged for Ron to go to a Day Centre, specially geared for dementia patients, twice a week. At first this was in a hospital, where they watched Ron and gave numerous tests to find out if there was more that could be done for him. Then he went to a very pleasant home run by the Salvation Army. He fitted in better there. The amusements arranged at the hospital were just not Ron's type at all. He would come home with his pockets full of bingo numbers and some of the old songs, all carefully written out by hand for him to join in. But he was no singer, and hated these times. I must say that he soon reached the stage where no entertainment would work. I am full of admiration for the staff of every home and centre he went to, they did an admirable job.

When the ambulance called in the morning to take him away for the day I heaved a sigh of utter relief. Eileen and I cleaned rooms, and did the washing, changed the beds and prepared several meals in advance, almost wearing ourselves out.

Then we set off to get a glimpse of the sea, or to visit the shops, knowing that Ron was well looked after for a few hours. This meant that we only had to work out a programme for Ron five days of the week. It took some doing!

The garden at Little Torch had no secure gate, but was, back and front, very "open plan" in design. This is one of the pleasant features of the house, but it proved a very difficult problem for us as Ron's endeavours to wander became more frequent.

He became quite adept at slipping past us and making for the door. One day I was working in the kitchen, and didn't notice him as he slipped by, opened the front door and was gone. I detected an unusual draught, and discovered the door wide open, and no sign of Ron. I called out but there was no answer. He wasn't in the garden, so I tried the main house, where the visitors were. I called at each bedroom door, for I had once found him standing in a bedroom wondering how to get out. There was no sight or sound of Ron, so I came to the conclusion that he had gone farther afield.

As the time went by and he had not appeared, I shuddered at the thought of the busy road at the end of the drive, and wondered what could have happened to him. Then I looked out of the window and saw, appearing over the little incline in the driveway, the shapes of three people walking towards the house. Oh the relief! Yes! There was Ron, with a kind lady either side of him, coming up the drive like a triumphant hero! Our dear Dorothy, "The little old lady at the end of the drive", had found Ron wandering in among the traffic and, with her friend, had brought him home.

We were not able to completely secure any of the doors against someone getting out, so we just had to be vigilant. Later that same day, Eileen was ironing in the hallway when Ron crept by without being seen, and went off again. This time we didn't discover it straightaway, and as the daylight was gradually waning, the matter took on some urgency. I phoned Dorothy, but she was out. Eileen went for a walkabout to look for Ron, but came back having seen no-one who had met up with him.

I felt I had to phone the police, as the light was going by now. The police were so very kind, and assured me that they would do something to find him. Then, as I was still speaking to them, the heads of five people appeared coming over the incline in the drive. "Just a minute!" I said to the police constable, "Some people are coming up the drive!"

"Right," he said. "I'll hold on until you are quite sure if one of them is your husband." I watched as they came into full view. Yes, there he was! Oh, how glad I was to see him! He was smiling all over his face, obviously pleased with himself, with his escort of FOUR ladies this time. I got the distinct impression he would have liked to go out again and try to get six escorts! The police constable couldn't have been more helpful, and assured me that I was to call any time I was worried. The whole episode, although it emphasized our problem as we coped with Ron's restlessness, made me so aware of the love and helpfulness with which we were surrounded.

There were several kind people who would take Ron for a short walk to try to while away the time. I saw them as angels in disguise, and thanked my heavenly Father for sending them. Eileen was specially helpful, and would walk the slow pace to which Ron's walking had deteriorated, time and time again, when he was particularly restless. How we sighed for a secure garden in which he could wander to his heart's content! It brought home to us the need we had for the right housing as the months went by, and we had nothing in sight to which we could move.

It was evident that we had to organise some sort of activity for the afternoons, which seemed to be the time when the wanderlust was at its height. The personality change in Ron hit me hard when we were planning these outings. He had always been so unselfish, so longing to give pleasure rather than have pleasure of his own. What a difference there was now! "Oh Lord," I cried, "do help me. I've completely lost the one I have loved and walked with for these 56 years!"

I joined the Alzheimer's Society, and although I never did manage to get to any of their meetings, I found their literature very helpful, and learned a few helpful hints when thinking of how to ease this restlessness. I read of others who had the same problèm, and how they were having to constantly remind themselves that there had been a complete character change in each person as the illness developed.

But there was no doubt that the greatest source of comfort for me at this time was from my Shepherd. He could be with me always! He didn't even sleep, and knew the agony of the night-time as well as the problems of the day. If I felt too tired to pray, too weary to frame words, or even think, I was sure of His love, and His tender provision. My Shepherd was with me THROUGH IT ALL.

It was good to have Eileen's help as we planned the afternoon outings. There were times when Ron's exasperating behaviour would have made me dissolve into tears, but one look at Eileen's face and I began to see the funny side of so much that happened.

We tried to take Ron to a llama farm which was reasonably near. He had always loved animals, and was so gentle with them. We went in, and saw tables set ready for afternoon tea. He refused to go any further until he had been given a cup of tea, though it was very early in the afternoon. After the tea we went to see the llamas. We hoped he would be interested, as they looked at us with their beautiful, expressive eyes, asking to be loved.

"Silly cows!" he snorted in disgust, "they've got long necks!" It became a family joke afterwards, and even now when we visit the farm, we remember the disdain with which he regarded these "silly cows". Nothing would interest him that day except a group of ladies who were spinning the fleeces into wool.

He didn't talk any sense to them, but they humoured him, and made him feel satisfied. I've never been able to thank those ladies, but I did appreciate their instinctive gentleness as they answered the most weird questions!

One day, we decided that a ride in the car might help Ron to calm down. But he refused to get into the car. "No," he kept saying, "I want to go into the other door." We took him to the other side of the car. No, that was not right. Then we realised that he wanted to get into the driving seat! He became angry when we had to say no, so I took him for a short walk down the drive, and tried to show him that I loved him. After a seven-minute walk he had calmed down, and was willing to get into the car, though NOT in the driving seat.

When we went to the seaside, the sun was either too hot, or the wind too cold, or he didn't want to walk because his feet hurt. A chiropodist had thoroughly inspected his feet and found nothing at all to cause discomfort. We decided it must be that at certain times he felt pain and discomfort more intensely, even when there was no apparent cause.

One day we went to Wakehurst Place, a beautiful National Trust property with delightful gardens. "Dad has always loved gardens, so let's borrow a wheelchair and show him round without him having to walk."

An elderly gentleman came forward to help us with the

wheelchair. Previously, when Ron had gone away to a nursing home the carer had tried to sit him in a wheelchair, and he had stubbornly refused to get into it. Nothing would make him sit in that flimsy thing! What would happen now? We held our breath! Ron took one look at the wheelchair and said, "I'm NOT going to sit in that thing!"

"But it is a very nice wheelchair," we began.

"No!" he replied, very definitely.

I would like to thank that gentleman in charge of wheelchairs at Wakehurst Place for his tact and patience. Ever so gently, he soothed Ron, and we were gradually able to get him to bend sufficiently to sit down. What a relief! We toured round the gardens, and although Ron didn't seem to be interested, there was a more contented look on his face. Mind you, Eileen had aching muscles in her arms for several days afterwards as she had pushed up-hill and down-dale so that Ron could see the beauty of the gardens.

At this time, Ron would spend a lot of his day, when not sleeping, walking round the house, and asking the same questions, "Why don't you go to the shop and get the tickets?"

"What tickets, dear?" I asked.

"The tickets to take us home," he wailed.

"But, this is home!" I said. "Look, you remember buying this suite, and that picture was the one we bought on our Silver Wedding day." I pointed out other memories of the past which were all around, but nothing would satisfy him.

"This is NOT home! I want you to take me home!"

# Through It All

As we were looking out for a new home I thought this was in his mind, and might have unsettled him, but I have discovered that many people with dementia and Alzheimer's problems wander round and ask to go home. The extent to which they suffer with disorientation is hard to understand, but it must be dreadful to feel constantly that you are in a foreign environment.

In our journey through the valley this next phase was the worst as the disorientation began to involve his personal needs as well as his mobility.

I was greatly helped by a chorus which I often sang to myself:

"Through it all, through it all,
I have learned to follow Jesus,
I have learned to trust in God.
Through it all, through it all,
I have learned to depend upon His Word."

And His word to me was still, "Though I pass through the valley of death, I will fear no evil, for THOU ART WITH ME, Thy rod and Thy staff they comfort me!"

# Chapter 9
## Agony And Angels

Agony and Angels - it would be impossible for me to separate the two. Agony, yes; it was deep and searing at times; but always, yes, always, there were Angels, if only we opened our eyes enough to see them. So, in this chapter I try to combine the two, because that is exactly how it happened!

I wanted to miss out this stage in our experience, but I knew I couldn't. We had already discovered that our dear beloved Ron was "not there" any more. Instead, we had his shell, and as the days went by that shell became more and more difficult to cope with. It was as if we had a baby to deal with, only instead of the great hope and joy of training a baby in personal hygiene and in social skills, there was no chance of doing the simplest training, no hope, just endurance.

The worse physical thing I had to contend with was double incontinence. There was no awareness of where to perform bodily functions, and no amount of cajoling or training would get through. Ron had to be watched every moment, as he would never find his way to the bathroom alone, nor know what to do when he got there. Our bathroom was a long narrow room, and this made attending to him doubly difficult. How I dreaded it when he would stand up and mutter "toilet"! It was always the time when he was most angry. I am sure that a little of his brain was working enough to let him feel frustration and humiliation at these times.

However, it did get very hard to cope with. "Just stand still for a minute dear until I fix the pad", would inevitably be the signal for him to move around, and make such a lot more washing than was necessary. I remember on one occasion the battle was very fierce. Ron told me in no uncertain terms to go away and leave him. I held on for a few more minutes, but he became quite violent. In desperation, I did something I was so ashamed of later on. I said, "All right, if I'm not wanted, and if you won't let me help you, then I'm GOING!" I went out of the door and locked it.

As I stood outside I felt overcome with guilt. What had I done? I turned instinctively to the Lord, Who knew all about it. Strength came into me, and with it, a tender love for this poor afflicted shell which used to be my dear one. I opened the door. He was standing as I had left him, not really aware that I had locked him in. But the anger had died in him, and I was in a calmer frame of mind. I managed to get him comfortable at last.

I am not a nurse, my forte is far more with writing and organising. I found the physical side of nursing Ron terribly hard. I felt sick from morning till night, and not at all interested in food. I felt I'd never get rid of the smell of illness, though Eileen and I completely scoured the whole flat every day, and actually it smelt very sweet and wholesome to others. I write this confession because I am absolutely sure that many carers suffer agonies of remorse over small things which upset them to the point of wanting to go away. I can only say that my only escape was as I turned to my Shepherd, and felt His loving power come into me and help me through.

By this time I had to persuade Ron to abandon his suits, shirts and ties, which he had always worn, even on holiday, and to introduce him to track suits. This was a hard thing for him to accept, another loss of dignity, which even in his deteriorating state, he did feel I am sure. The family and friends rallied round and we were able to get some very nice trousers and tops so that he always looked well turned out, and it was so much easier to wash such informal wear than the more traditional clothing. In fact, all this time, when Ron had to depend so utterly on others to wash him, clothe him and lead him, must have been dreadful for any awareness left in him.

Ron had lost the consciousness of time a long time ago, and was fast losing the sense of where he was. He would start to undress without warning in the hallway, lounge or anywhere else, and at other times would go to bed fully dressed if we didn't keep a check on him. One day, I had put his clothing out ready for when he woke up, but had not put it on his bed. I went to prepare the dinner, when the door opened and he came out of the bedroom wearing my clothes. He had gone to my drawer and enjoyed himself having a grand time choosing what to wear. He was wearing my skirt as a sort of shawl, one of his legs was through my jumper sleeves, and he had decked himself round his shoulders with my underwear. I just had to disappear for a moment and laugh before I sorted him out.

But angels were there! Michael would never call himself an angel, but his firm yet loving words, greeting each new day, were so looked forward to. It was a great miss when he had well-earned time off! "Come on Ron, my lad," he would say, trying to get some response from Ron's sleeping form. "No, Ron, oh no!" he would say, "don't do that!" when Ron seemed to be behaving badly. Yet he was always so calm and level-headed. I was very glad that he was able to appreciate the way Ron behaved with me at times, and was able to understand my problems so clearly. We could talk together about little things which I wondered if Ron needed help with, and he was always so constructive with his advice. Yes, Eileen and I looked forward to Michael's visits eagerly.

Then there was David, who managed to persuade Ron to have a bath, very much against his will! David made it such fun that I could actually hear Ron laughing at times when they were splashing around in the bathroom. David always had a smile on his face, and was the first person outside the family who helped Ron to come to terms with receiving help with personal care.

I must tell you, too, about Peter. He came from the organisation "Crossroads" and what a blessing his coming was. He would take Ron out for a walk, sit with him in the recreation ground, talk about all sorts of things, often with no response. He would fix up a clothes-line which had broken, bring in some shopping, and cheer us up as we had our coffee together – though Peter drank only water!

Other angels came along too, in the shape of white-clad carers who helped to get Ron ready for bed, and also attended him each weekend. All of them were so different, and had their own individual ways of encouraging, but they all had a real love for the work they were doing.

I was now living in a world of incontinence pads, kylie sheets and things I didn't know even existed a year ago. Special protective wear, bottles and waterproofs were articles belonging to a foreign world to me. But the statutory services were at my side helping with these things, always ready to go as far as they could to alleviate my load, as well as keeping a caring eye on Ron. They were severely hampered by financial restrictions; it was so sad to see them fighting to get supplies which should have been more readily available. I saw them as God's provision for me, and I felt decidedly cherished as a carer, which made the grim side of it all the easier to bear.

Meanwhile, we were living through each day trying to cope with the difficulties. Some of the books told me to try to divert Ron from himself. "Try going through a photo album and talking about the old days," it advised. But it didn't work with Ron, after all, he was never keen on photographs when all was well! TV, even Christian videos and lovely hymn-singing only seemed to aggravate him. He lived for meal-times, and that word which struck terror into my soul, "toilet"!

I discovered how badly affected Ron was by flickering lights, and any undue noise. He began to have hallucinations too at this time, sure that someone else was around and convinced that we should be able to see them too.

We had very few visitors. I used to stand at the window sometimes and see friends of long-standing calling at the house next door, and not thinking, or not daring, I don't know which, to come in and say 'Hello'. Some of my family found it very hard to come. Some didn't come at all, and how I longed for them to see me. But there were angels even here, and Liz, our eldest granddaughter came and tried hard to help Grandad to have some pleasure. It worked at first very well, but there came a day when she dropped in to see us, and Grandad didn't even recognise her. I could see the hurt in her face, though she didn't let it stay there, knowing full well that it simply meant that Grandad had lost even more of his brain. It is surprising how well some people cope and how badly others do. Some of my friends did not seem able to come to terms with the problem. Dear Sandy coped better than most, in fact, she managed to get through to Ron even after I had failed to do so. I felt I wanted to go out and ask people to come in and talk to us about ordinary things, anything to take us out of this sordid saga of sickness and dying. One or two did come, and they were like angels to us.

Just one thing would make an impression on Ron for five minutes at the most, and that was if I read a portion of Scripture to him. It would bring a response immediately, though the power of concentration would not be there for long.

There were other things which had to be dealt with as well. Ron had for some time been unable to sign his name. It is amazing how many times we need to sign things. So we had to obtain an enduring power of attorney so that I could manage his affairs completely. What a topsy-turvey world I felt I was living in! From being a very loved and cherished wife, who was never allowed to have any money worries, suddenly I was moving in a nightmare situation with the requirements of modern living where everything had to be signed and sealed!

I have mentioned "the little old lady at the bottom of the drive", as Ron used to call her. She was an angel indeed, and always there if I needed her. Also, when Eileen was taking a well-deserved holiday, I had angels in the shape of my brother Bernard and his wife Mavis. They came at a time when I was desperate and all alone. The incontinence was particularly difficult to cope with, and I was utterly exhausted. They were ready to be wakened at night, if I was having a bad time with Ron, and were very willing to take me out when Ron was at the day centre, so that I could look at any suitable houses for sale. I remember them standing, as I was trying to deal with a difficult occasion with Ron, and saying, "Stella, you CAN'T carry on like this, it is far too much for anyone. Something must be done!" It made me start to consider what I could do to get through the physical difficulties which were getting worse.

Other people came along too. There was Len, who helped us for a few weeks, and Barbara, who filled in for a few days when I was alone. And always, consistently, there was Eileen, or Edith, as Ron insisted on calling her. She was always there, anticipating needs and praying with me every day, which was such a strength. Yes, I had my share of angels, without doubt.

Some would-be helpers found it hard to come to terms with the change in someone they had such deep respect for. They battled with their feelings and came through to be angels in spite of how they felt. Others didn't manage quite so well. But we thank the Lord for all who tried.

I mustn't forget my family who gave me all the time they could manage, and Gail and Alan who lived in Little Torch. They were true neighbours, and lived through many a crisis with me. The doctor, too, was a tower of strength, and cared enough to call or phone at the slightest development of the illness. The Lord certainly does give His angels charge over His children. They helped me over many rough places in the journey through the valley.

# Through It All

Cutting the cake — Where shall I start?

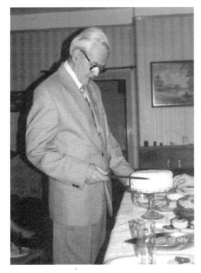

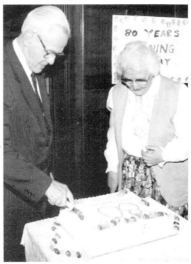

80 years and still going strong! (1995)

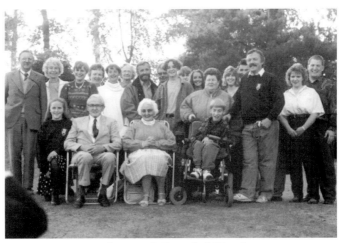

Grandma and Grandad Heath —
Golden Wedding Anniversary 1993

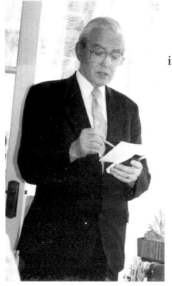

At a Keswick Houseparty
We hosted houseparties at
Convention time for visually
impaired people for over 30 years

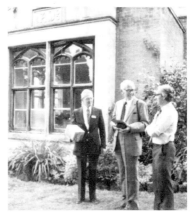

Chatting with Mr Gladstone
Moore and Ray Adams
outside the library

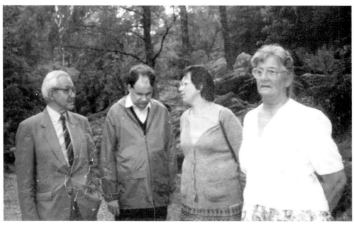

Walking in the Lake District with some of the members of the
Torch Houseparty at Keswick

# Chapter 10
## Home?... Where?

All the time, when the trauma of Ron's illness was taking its course, we were aware of mounting anxiety about where we would be living.

There was no question. We would not be able to stay where we were, not only because it was so unsuitable for us while we were nursing Ron, but because the flat was needed, in view of the developments which were vital to the work at Little Torch. The whole domestic area had to be scraped out and new plumbing and electrics installed, as well as a lot of structural alterations long overdue. It would be quite impossible for Gail and Alan and the children to live in their rooms in the main house, yet it was important that they should be "on-site" to keep an eye on the progress of the work. There was no real pressure put upon us, though we were aware that the workmen were scheduled to start in mid-December.

The door had closed for us to have any help from Torch itself; indeed, not knowing this, we had earlier negotiated for a house in Crawley which could have been made suitable. However, when we realised there was no money available to buy it, we had to withdraw, and the house was sold to someone else.

The months were slipping by, and it was now September, and nothing was in view. We had worked out the accommodation we felt we needed for Ron and Eileen and myself. We had a certain amount of Torch stocks of literature and books, and an increasing amount of equipment which was the property of the work of Shalom Christian Outreach, the new ministry which supported

Sandy in her role as the Singing Evangelist. We felt we needed to have a downstairs bedroom in an annex of some sort, a small office, and upstairs accommodation which Eileen could use entirely for herself. Two things were needed, one was to find the right property, and the other was to have the money with which to buy it.

The way the money was found still fills me with wonder, and makes me want to glorify God every day of my life! Finding myself up against the problems, and being unable to share them with Ron, I turned to my dear prayer partners who had stood by us through many trials over the years. I sent them a letter telling them of our need of a home. I didn't ask for money at all, but thanked those who had sent to us. "Please pray for me," I asked, "I don't know just what to do."

The result was staggering! From far and near, from people I knew well and others who I knew less, came gifts "For your new home". And the beautiful cards, texts, and messages of encouragement melted me to tears every day when the post came. What love! How humble it made me feel! I could see this was something very big which the Lord had ordered, so we set up a trust so that the money would be wisely dealt with. It was not long before the trustees announced that we had enough to start house-hunting seriously.

Our first thought was to go back to look in the Crawley area, to see if there was something suitable there. There seemed to be nothing at all! Copthorne was tried next, then Horsham. We began to wonder if there would be anywhere suitable for us.

Then one day in September, "quite by chance", though with such a wonderful Good Shepherd how could anything be "by chance", we saw a property advertised in a paper which sounded as if it had all we needed. It was in East Grinstead, which we had never even thought of choosing. We made arrangements to see it. It was amazing how right it was! There was a little office already fitted with shelves and plugs suitable for the computer, there was a cosy lounge opening on to a really lovely patio, the kitchen was just a dream to me after the little galley kitchen in the annex at Hurstpierpoint. The fitments were there for spices and magnetic knife racks, and ample storage space. It was every woman's dream! We only had to replace the cooker, and nothing else was essential to be done. We could move straight in! And yes, there was an annex, opening on to the patio, with access through the kitchen, bright windows overlooking the garden, and a little en suite shower and toilet, it was just perfect!

Eileen, too, was very happy. There were four rather small bedrooms, but they suited Eileen very well, and she was overcome with joy when she saw the bath. Evidently, she had prayed for one special thing, a long bath! And there it was, absolutely made to measure! The trustees got busy with all the necessary surveys and reports, and eventually, in October, we were able to purchase the house. There is one thing which is sure, from first to last we could see the hand of God in our house-moving plans.

Since those days we have discovered a wealth of Christian friendship and fellowship in East Grinstead, and can only worship the Lord humbly for His care and love, and the sure way He has led us! It was not surprising that after all this the completion date was just in time – the middle of December!

We started straightaway packing boxes whenever we could on those days when Ron was at the Day Centre. It would have confused him if he had seen us doing that before it was absolutely necessary.

However, Ron was still deteriorating all the time, and the way was getting harder as we tried to cope with him. What steps should I be taking to secure somewhere really right for dear Ron? It was evident that we would have to find him a permanent care home before too long.

The senior social worker and the doctor had already pressed our claim to get financial help to place Ron in a nursing home, but each time the request had reached the committee it had been turned down.

Alyson, my intrepid daughter-in-law, was galvanised into action!

"Mother," she said, "you must write to the chairman of this committee that is blocking the way and arrange to go and see him!"

I began to shake at the knees. That was not me! I could never think what to say when faced with officials like that. "Don't you worry at all," she said, " I'm coming with you, and I'll tell them a thing or two!"

The chairman was very gracious, and welcomed us to his office, though we had been told that he NEVER received visits of this sort. He listened attentively whilst we put our case. He said, "It is obvious you should never be left to cope with this situation. Your husband's condition is way beyond what can be treated at home. He needs to be taken into a nursing home which deals with these special needs. But, there are so many other cases which need this help, and I'm not sure how soon your case could be settled, maybe in January, if you are lucky."

"That's impossible," said Alyson, "Mother has to move out of her present home by the middle of December, so they need something to be done before then. What can you do about that?"

The kind man rubbed his chin. "Well," he said, thoughtfully, "Mrs Heath here will obviously not be able to manage to tackle a move and continue to care for her husband at the same time."

"So, where do we go from here?" said Alyson, determined to get an answer.

"There is one thing I can do," he replied. "I can give you authority to extend the temporary respite care which is usually arranged for carers. As you know, this amounts to a week's respite every six weeks. As the situation is obviously very urgent, you can use the respite care for as long as you need it, in any nursing home which we recognise. It is not the same as being given a permanent placement I know, but it might help you through this time."

We said a heartfelt "Thank you", feeling very glad of such an offer.

Alyson and I had previously done a tour of eight or nine nursing homes which took patients needing EMI care. Some of them didn't seem right for father, but there were a few which we could imagine him settling in as well as could be expected. One of these was in the village of Cowfold where Alyson worked as Head Teacher. It was in a rural setting, with a view of trees, squirrels, pheasants and many birds from the window. We arranged for father to go there towards the end of November, when we would have to seriously pack up and prepare to move.

We had visited another home, which was just beautiful. The atmosphere was so full of love and of the presence of the Lord. I felt a real bond with the Sister in charge. However, there was no vacancy, and we would have to put Ron's name down and wait for a place, which might be a long time. I have such warm memories of our visit there, but obviously it could not be of use to us over the period of the move. The Sister wrote to me several times; she was one of those who encouraged me to write about our experiences, as she saw so many people shattered by the problems of dementia and Alzheimer's disease.

Then, one Monday evening, before Ron was due to go into the Cowfold Nursing Home for a fortnight, I noticed a further deterioration in him. He was not eating or drinking properly, and so I phoned the doctor. He came straightaway and prescribed some pills to help. Eileen went straight out to find a chemist's shop which was open. I was left alone with Ron. He had slept a lot that evening, but he woke up, and decided to change his seat, moving across to the settee, where he promptly went to sleep again.

Later, one of the young carers came to put Ron to bed.

"Hello Ronald, I've come to put you to bed!" she said cheerfully. There was no response, only a raising of the head. So I sat beside Ron and tried to help him to wake up sufficiently to walk to the bedroom. But he wouldn't or couldn't stand up. We had known times when he had not stood up to go to the bedroom as a form of protest, but I was not at all sure what was the matter this time. The little nurse had a schedule of other people waiting to be put to bed, so I felt I ought to try to encourage Ron to move if possible. It took us half an hour to get him across the lounge and into the hall. Suddenly, he raised his voice and shouted, "Stella, what are you doing to me?" I was shocked at the vehemence in his tone, and wondered what I had done wrong. That phrase was the last intelligible word he said to me!

After a few more shuffled steps, Ron collapsed in a heap in the hall. Being wise after the event, I should have phoned for an ambulance, but I could only think of getting Ron comfortably in bed. So, instead, I ran next door to Gail. Bless her, she came straightaway, picked Ron up and carried him on to the bed, just as easily (it seemed) as picking up a teddy bear. We were able to get Ron comfortable after that.

The next day he was very subdued, but the carer was able to wash and dress him without any trouble. He didn't speak to me any more, and only said the minimum to anyone else. Eating was poor, drinking difficult, and communication was nil. The doctor came and made immediate arrangements for Ron to be taken to the nursing home by ambulance, as we would never have managed to get him into a car.

Even then the angels were busy! The nurse in charge of the ambulance was a radiant Christian, and we were able to chat to each other on the journey. Also, we had two dear long-standing friends who arrived to visit us on the very day when Ron was taken to the nursing home. They were such a cheer, even making Ron smile.

What a relief it was to know that Ron would be having expert attention, and a lot of love and care as well. The staff at Homelands had enjoyed having him on his last visit, and had declared that he had made a lasting impression on one rather difficult man by his kindness and gentle example. This man had been easier to manage since Ron's visit. I was amazed and so glad to hear that! He might be rough with me, but he was still a precious child of God, and had lived with that lovely link with Christ for so long. It was good that even when part of him was dying, he could still pass on some of that spiritual quality which had been so evident in his life.

During that next week, Ron went downhill fast. Phil, our son, who lives in Bridgwater, phoned to say he felt strongly that he should come up to see father. He picked up his sister Rosemary, and then they called for me. So, on that Friday morning we three were sitting in Ron's room, drinking the tea so thoughtfully provided. Ron seemed to be asleep. He had not eaten or drunk anything much, but lay there, sleepily waiting for the call to go to his Lord. Then the door opened and Alyson came in. "I've got a few moments," she said, "so I felt I must come!" About ten minutes later Ron's breathing changed. Rosemary ran to get the Sister, and they arrived back just as our dear Ron was breathing his last.

It was at once a sad, yet happy occasion. How could we wish him back in that old worn-out body! Yet we were already missing his love and counsel. Now it had gone for ever.

Ron did not make it to the earthly home we were moving to in East Grinstead, and he didn't have to spend long in a nursing home either. We knew so surely now he had truly gone home to the place which his Shepherd had been preparing for him, in heaven. The One who met him at Bruges and said, "I did it for you", was there now waiting to receive him. Ron had been so grateful for the way his Saviour had died for him, to cleanse him from sin, and made him His own child. Now he had arrived to spend eternity in His presence. Ron looked so peaceful, truly at rest at last. There cannot be the same depth of sorrow and despair when we watch a precious child of God go home!

Up at Hallaton, the Torch Council was meeting. The subject for discussion was whether or not they should go forward in faith and refurbish Little Torch so that it would meet government standards. It was a question of vital importance, because, if they said that they were not going to take this step, then Little Torch would have to close, and the work cease. The door opened, and a voice said, "Dad Heath has gone to be with Christ." There was silence for some minutes, then one of them said, "I don't think there is any doubt that Dad Heath would have said we had to go ahead in faith with this project!" They all agreed.

The refurbishments have taken place, and there is a lovely quiet garden beside the chapel where Dad's ashes were laid to rest under the sundial. The garden has plants and trees provided by members of the family. It is good to know that his remains are where he spent so many happy years of service.

Why did Dad Heath have to go to Glory this way? I don't know the answer, but I am sure that through the darkest times we have found a deeper trust in our Shepherd than we ever had before. Such lessons are eternal.

We asked for no flowers except from the family. Instead, we suggested gifts in Ron's memory to help forward the work in Malawi which was always dear to him. Over £3,000 was given, and has been used to house the Christian beggars whose lot was so dreadful, and also to help establish the braille printing work on the compound in Blantyre.

Have I any regrets? Yes, I have one or two. I wish I had understood more the pain and bewilderment which Ron had to go through, though I'm not sure I could have done anything more to help him. I also have taken some time to come to terms with the last words Ron said to me. Friends have spoken of the lovely messages which their loved ones have given as they died, I didn't have anything like that. But I can look back at many times of sweet fellowship when times were easier, and I know so surely that Ron is joyful in his Heavenly Home, and I am happily settled in my earthly one, with a few more years of service before me, God-willing.

David the Psalmist said, "Surely goodness and mercy shall follow me all the days of my life, and I will dwell in the house of the Lord forever." Goodness and mercy have been likened to two faithful sheepdogs, following us all the way. I couldn't always see them, but, as I look back and see the way I've been led, I realise that they have followed me. I can appreciate so clearly now how good, and how merciful, God has been to us all. I really do love that 23$^{rd}$ Psalm.

A wonderful thanksgiving service was held for Ron soon after his death. Many people, including a large contingent from Torch, came from long distances to share in praise for his life. At that service so much praise was offered to the Lord in all that was said and sung. It was good to have a tribute from the family, voiced by Phil, and to hear Gordon, who has been our friend for so long, reminiscing about Torch in the early days. Charlotte, our youngest granddaughter, read the scripture, Sandy sang very movingly "Face to face with Christ my Saviour", and the rest of the family stood beside me and formed a veritable choir as we sang some of Dad's favourite hymns. Karen, another granddaughter, read the poem which I felt the Lord gave me on the occasion of Ron's entry to Glory. There were other tributes as well, and the whole event was a powerful testimony to Ron's consistent life.

What a glorious end to a traumatic year! How true to life this is when we are walking with the Lord. There is always a victorious end to each battle. Thank God for His Shepherd-care. How do people get by in life without Him? How much He longs to help them too. "Come to Me all who are weary and heavy-laden, and I will give you rest," said Jesus in Matthew 11:28. Surely that is a verse specially written for carers.

# I'VE GOT A NEW HOME!

Turn out the cupboards, the disarray,
All of the rubbish, which every day
Has piled in the corners, and cluttered our way,
Relics of time which is passing away,
For I've got a new home.

Out of the mists of our earth-bound life,
With all its battles, pain and strife,
I'm off to a new and glorious place,
No sin, and no sorrow – and all of God's grace,
I've got a new home.

None of our rubbish can move with us there,
No bitterness, darkness, no sin, no despair,
Only a new-born and beautiful soul
Washed from defilement, made perfectly whole,
In God's new home.

Surely and certainly we each will receive
The Call to eternity. To those who believe,
"Come now, blessed children, there's a place just for you
In the glory of heaven, where all things are new."
I've got a new home!

But say, when the call comes, suppose all we hear
Is a sad and dark greeting when we get there.
"Depart, I don't know you – you can't bring earth's toys
Into this beautiful home of all joys.
No room in my home!"

Lord, help us to value those treasures above
Which You are now offering to us in Your love.
To check on our values, choose the riches that last,
When the baubles of earth-life are broken and past.
For we're going home.

Brussels in 1998

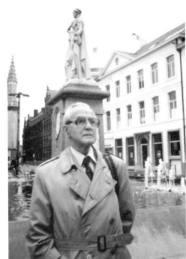

The trip to Belgium
where Ron had a special
blessing at Bruges in 1998

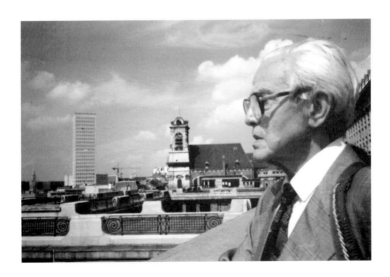

Enjoying a joke
with Sandy

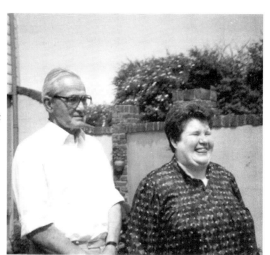

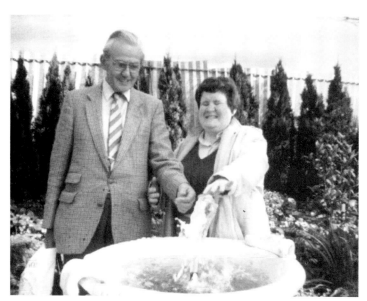

"Come on Sandy, you can feel this one"
Dad Heath had the knack of helping blind people to explore
their environment

# Chapter 11
## Grieving

Grieving! "Don't be afraid to grieve," my dear friends kept saying to me.

At first I was numb, like a zombi, doing all that was necessary when faced with a bereavement. The funeral arrangements, taking the death certificates to places I had never visited before, were all done on auto-pilot; so was the arranging for the Thanksgiving Service and notifying friends of the passing of Ron.

The zombi stage lasted well over Christmas and the New Year. Probably that was as well, as these happy family times can be difficult for those who are recently bereaved.

Then came the remembrances. At first, all I could think of was the sordid and sad, the problems, the pain of his remarks made in anger, though never meant by the true Ron. The smell of sickness was still with me, and the routine of the sick room, pills and ointments, the stress of trying to keep everything clean and hygienic were vividly remembered. There was a measure of relief in the memory, as I gradually came to realise that this respite was not just for a week, but for ever. Now it was all in the past, and I must move on from it. But, as I let go of those memories, I found it more painful.

I forgot Ron, the invalid, and remembered the loving, upright, caring man he really was. The sense of loss became more intense, and it took some time and effort to cope with it. Even now, when I am reading a book aloud to some of my blind friends, I find myself dissolving into tears when a particularly powerful paragraph or tender emotion is portrayed.

"Don't be afraid of grieving," my kind friends said. I could add, "Indeed, but make sure you hold fast to Jesus, the One Who fully understands. He alone can turn your mourning into joy."

There were difficulties socially, too, at times. I had always been part of US, as Ron and I were known as "one". Now, I was just poor, little, insignificant ME, a widow, a relict, as they used to be called. It seems to be easier to entertain couples, for couples fit easily into the social scene when planning parties. I found it hard at first to cope with this "lost, spare part" feeling when mixing with others, even though people went out of their way to be helpful. Maybe this was the price I had to pay for the way Ron and I had moved around so much together.

Loneliness crept in too. How lonely it can be, even in a crowd. Laughter and friendly banter can bring on the beginnings of "poor old me" – something to reject immediately as nothing but a hindrance to all that is good. I would go to the shops and spot a real bargain, "three for the price of one!" and just what we needed! I'd come home wanting to share my "find" with Ron, but he was no longer there. It was the same with happy events, exciting news and funny things. For some time I couldn't get away from the bubbling excitement of wanting to share them with Ron. When writing letters I couldn't at first get used to putting the personal pronoun singular, and kept writing "we"! Our togetherness was very precious, and I think it is meaning more to me now, as I discover the gap there is in my life without Ron.

Then there are times when problems have to be sorted out. I don't know what to do sometimes, and so I have to try to relate to others, and trust their judgement and advice. The trouble is that no-one can fully take the place of my dear one – only God. But how real and precious His company is at times like this.

I understand a little more now the instructions which were written in the early Church about needing to care for widows. Times and needs are different but these days can be very bewildering for those left to cope alone. Perhaps the attitude shown in the Acts needs to be encouraged in today's fast-moving society. Thank the Lord for places where there is so much love and understanding. Widows need it.

I realised that I had to step out and do something different. I still had my writing, which I love, and also personal contact with my blind friends, but I felt I must find another way to express myself. The answer came when I took a Water Colour Painting Course at Ashburnham Place. I'm by no means a genius, but I have found myself studying the world around me in a new way. The light and shade which makes a good picture is there all around us, and it takes both to make it lifelike. How true this is in our experience. We need to have light and shade, joy and sorrow, to grow into balanced maturity. There are truly many treasures of darkness which are revealed to us in our "valley" experiences. This new outlet helped me considerably as I passed through my grieving.

There are still some small, innocent remarks or events which can open the floodgates of grief, but these occasions are becoming more rare as I go forward into all that my Shepherd has for me.

Jesus experienced grief in its most acute form when He was forsaken on the Cross, taking my place and bearing the penalty for my sin. "My God, my God, why have You forsaken me?" He cried. How lovely to remember that this was not the end, but the joy of resurrection followed three days later. Sorrow and joy, it is the pattern of life here on earth. But, because Jesus suffered the loneliness of being forsaken by His Father for me, I can be confident that He will never forsake me, but be with me all my days. That means a lot to those who grieve.

"Weeping may endure for a night, but joy comes in the morning!" Psalm 30:5.

# Chapter 12
## Caring

Carers! There are so many of them! Young and old, they minister day after day to people in physical need. Some of those cared for seem unable to show gratitude for all the help they are given, others have sweet grateful dispositions, and are a delight to minister to.

But all carers, especially those who are involved in caring full-time, have one thing in common, they carry a constant, unremitting burden of care. Spare a thought and a prayer for the carers. Sometimes, they will be looking out of the window, as I did, at the busy world outside and long for someone from that world to call and say a cheery "Hello, how are you?"

I remember feeling so desolate when I heard hearty laughter coming from the house next door, and having to fight a major battle with "poor old me"!

Just a handshake, a few minutes to chat, even a cuddle as appropriate, would have meant so much to me at that time. It would have helped me to feel a person again, instead of a piece of household equipment devoted to the smooth running of the establishment, and the welfare of the patient.

Some people did call, and brought news of the friends I knew; refreshing conversations, jokes, joy and laughter, what a relief these visitors brought. The little world inside the home where sickness reigns becomes so small, so limited. Thank God for friends and relatives who take the trouble to visit the carers as well as the sick. Such friends are worth their weight in gold.

There is a growing awareness of the need of carers. For carers are people too, and their number is increasing daily as more and more people need to be cared for. So many carers go under because of the many stresses which come their way. I was very encouraged and helped by the way people like nurses and social workers, and the people from organisations like Crossroads, showed real concern and understanding when coming alongside me.

Could more be done by churches to strengthen the faith and meet the spiritual need of those who are caring for others? The task these people are doing is valued by the Master who spoke so highly of those who give a cup of cold water in His Name. A ministry of "caring for carers". For those who are coping with dementia sufferers, this would be so welcome, for they too need to have help and care themselves.

But, in the final analysis, humans can only go so far in helping us through the valleys of life. The one great way of treading through the dark times is when we are in close touch with the Shepherd. I pray He will be very real and precious to all carers everywhere.

# Appendix

There are, apparently, three phases which people suffering from Alzheimer's or dementia go through.

The first is the failure of short-term memory, which also makes orientation difficult and causes the person to get lost even in familiar places. This gradually evolves until long-term memory is also affected.

The second period is infinitely more trying. The sufferer is aware of who he is and what he wants to do, but his brain finds it difficult to relay the messages to the rest of his body. Any instruction needs to be given several times for the simplest of jobs, and he has to be allowed time to make his legs work, or to start eating his meal. This gradually gets worse, until some messages are not transmitted to the body at all. The agony of the later stages of this phase are excruciating to watch. I wish I had been able to understand what was happening when Dad was going through this time, it might have helped me to be a greater support to him.

The last phase occurs when the brain is virtually dead, and even the natural functions are impaired until they stop altogether, and death comes as a blessed relief to sufferer and carer alike.

Helpful literature and support can be obtained from local benefits agency and social services – address in phone book.

Other sources of help are:

Alzheimer's Disease Society,
Gordon House,
10 Greencoat Place,
LONDON
SW1P 1PH
Tel. 020 7306 0606

Association of Crossroads Care Attendants Scheme,
10 Regent Place,
RUGBY
Warwickshire
CV21 2PN
Tel. 01788 573653

# Through The Valley Of Dementia

# Through It All